MW01702926

CHILDREN'S EYES

A Guide to Understanding

Dr. Judith Doctor

INFINITY
PUBLISHING.COM

Copyright © 2009 by Judith Doctor

All rights reserved. No part of this book shall be reproduced or transmitted in any form or by any means, electronic, mechanical, magnetic, photographic including photocopying, recording or by any information storage and retrieval system, without prior written permission of the publisher. No patent liability is assumed with respect to the use of the information contained herein. Although every precaution has been taken in the preparation of this book, the publisher and author assume no responsibility for errors or omissions. Neither is any liability assumed for damages resulting from the use of the information contained herein.

ISBN 0-7414-5706-7

Published by:

INFINITY
PUBLISHING.COM

1094 New DeHaven Street, Suite 100
West Conshohocken, PA 19428-2713
Info@buybooksontheweb. com
www. buybooksontheweb. com
Toll-free (877) BUY BOOK
Local Phone (610) 941-9999
Fax (610) 941-9959

Printed in the United States of America

Published December 2009

For my beloved husband and mentor
Daniel W. Doctor, M.D.

PREFACE

My story is rather straightforward – mother, pediatrician, eye physician and surgeon, and finally grandmother. During all my years restoring vision, maintaining good eye sight, preventing severe visual loss and even blindness, I discovered that most people do not understand eyes. They take for granted this wonderful, precious gift of nature. They abuse them, misuse them, and often neglect them. As long as a picture is clear before them when they open their eyes they do not routinely examine them. They squeeze, squint, and rearrange their face in order to avoid glasses, which might restore clearer vision. People choose non-medical resources rather than eye physicians. The special gift of eyesight is held with little regard until vision slips away. Eyes are fragile. Problems have to be detected early. An eye physician has no room for mistakes.

I discovered long ago that children have different vision problems than adults. Early detection of refractive and developmental growth changes can prevent blindness. I may have been the first ophthalmologist to establish a Pediatric Eye Clinic at Manhattan Eye Ear and Throat Hospital whose specific objective was to recognize and prevent eye problems in pre-school children. This clinic targeted the vulnerable group of babies, infants, and toddlers from birth to three years of age.

Parents have often asked me during their child's eye exam; where can I get more information about my child's eye condition? This book is designed to answer these questions, to enable parents, teachers, nurses and lay people to decide, is this a problem or not? Where should I go to get help? How soon must the problem be corrected? Is surgery indicated and at what age? Essentially within this handbook, I wish to establish a basic guide, a quick readable reference. This book is not a text book or course in Pediatric Ophthalmology. My desire is that the reader will gain greater insight and understanding of children's vision problems. This understanding will translate into early detection of serious potential vision loss and eventually prevent unnecessary blindness.

Before you read this handbook let me try to clear up the confusion that some people have about eye care providers. Here are the facts. An ophthalmologist, unfortunate word and difficult to pronounce, is an eye physician.

The word ophthalmos comes from the Greeks and means eyes. These doctors train as physicians by going to accredited medical schools and choose to devote their postgraduate years in an eye residency program which takes three years after medical school and internship. In addition many physicians go on to further training in fellowship programs which broaden their knowledge in areas such as cataract, cornea, glaucoma, retina, pediatric ophthalmology, eye plastics, neurophthalmology, strabismus, etc. During these years of training, eye physicians learn how to care for their patients both medically and surgically. Other eye care providers or optometrists are not medical doctors. Often the two professions are associated in one eye care practice. A patient who goes to an office for an eye exam should ask for and receive information regarding his or her provider's training and professional background. Eyes are too valuable to treat casually.

TABLE OF CONTENTS

CHAPTER I

VISION OF THE NEWBORN

The visual acuity of a normal neonate or newborn is approximately 20/400. This is true because the macula has not yet fully developed. The macula is the name given to the part of the retina we use to see objects and to read. Many have likened the eye to a camera. The lens of the eye focuses as a lens in the camera. The film of the camera is the retina of the eye. The macula is located in the retina at the back of the eye. The macula continues to mature as the infant grows. At birth, a normal infant can fixate or look at a light. When he follows the light, his eyes may appear jerky, not smooth. At approximately three months of age, his eyes move together evenly in one direction. When normal birth weight infants (greater than five pounds, eight ounces) are delayed in their ability to follow and fixate on light, one should rule out medical problems. By four months of age an infant can accommodate or focus and develop stereopsis or depth perception.

If necessary, a newborn can have a thorough eye exam. The eye physician is able to test for the existence of vision by means of a flashlight directed toward her eyes. The flashlight is moved from right to left or vice versa. The physician carefully observes this follow response. The physician carefully examines other parts of the eye as well.

She evaluates the cornea, or shiny part of the eye, the color of the iris, the size and movement of the pupil and the symmetry between the eyes. Symmetry and clarity of the eye are the most important features. In addition, clarity means that the corneas of both eyes must be perfectly clear.

At two to four months of age, parents should observe that their infant can follow puppets or a mobile placed above him. Most normal birth weight infants are slightly far sighted or have hyperopia. This may change as they mature, depending on their genetic inheritance and whether their family members wear glasses. The eye grows in stages. Children, whose families have a strong history of nearsightedness or myopia, should have their eyes examined at birth. This holds true for prematures who have a high risk of developing near sightedness. Prematures should be examined in the nursery prior to discharge from the hospital. Congenital myopia begins early. These babies can be refracted or examined for glasses with the aid of a retinoscope, an instrument which helps determine the power of the eye. There is no pain associated with this technique of examination. Most infants are cooperative. In order to perform a retinoscopy, the pupils are dilated. The physician uses a series of lenses and a hand held instrument to observe a reflex. If myopia is considered significant, glasses are usually prescribed regardless of the patient's age.

It is sometimes difficult for parents to recognize nearsightedness in their newborn, since most babies hold their toys close to them and look at objects as they bring them to their mouths. Severe myopia can cause sensory deprivation. The baby is less interested in her surroundings.

She often clings to her parents and is shy. Parents who are good observers can prevent behavior problems if they are able to recognize them as a possible sign of poor vision. Parents must be alerted to the possibility that shyness may be a result of poor vision. A proper eye exam is indicated.

CHAPTER II

VISUAL ASSESSMENT OF AN INFANT AND TODDLER

How does an eye physician assess the vision of an infant and toddler?

1. Infants with a normal birth weight history can be tested in the following manner:

   a) the physician notices if the infant turns to a light source, i.e., a window or flashlight;

   b) Does infant follow faces?

   c) Does infant cry when the indirect ophthalmoscope is used during examination?

   d) Does infant blink when light is directed toward him?

   e) A rotating drum can be used to gauge visual acuity in infants as young as two months of age, since the peripheral retina is mature enough to be stimulated by this time.

f) The physician creates nystagmus (involuntary movement of the eyes) by moving the drum in front of the infant's eye vertically and horizontally. The drum has black lines of different widths on a white field. The thickness of these lines presented and the child's positive response will be recorded by the physician and used to determine the approximate visual acuity of the patient.

2. Toddlers' vision is assessed essentially by giving parents "E" cards. The cards are sized and represent visual acuity levels on the Snellen Eye Chart. Parents are instructed to ask their children to point with their fingers the direction that the fingers of the "E" points, i.e., up, down, to the right, to the left. For children who have difficulty with eye-hand coordination, pictures can be substituted which correlate in size to the Snellen chart letters. Each eye is tested separately. Finally, if determination of visual acuity is difficult due to poor cooperation, it is best to make the first exam a "get acquainted with the doctor visit" and allow a friendship to develop between your child and the doctor. In most cases, when recording vision assessment is unsatisfactory, the pupils are dilated in order to perform a retinoscopy. The light used during this exam is not harmful to the child and the effect of the drop does not last long.

3. What does it mean when vision is not equal in both eyes? As previously stated, eyes are usually symmetrical. The finding of different vision, even if it only represents one line, is important. Many things must be considered:

   a) Amblyopia

   b) Medical problem(s) relating to the eyes

   c) Strabismus (misalignment of the eyes)

   d) Refractive problem(s)

CHAPTER III

INFLUENCES ON CHILDREN'S VISUAL OUTCOME

The term "Lazy Eye" commonly used by lay people to describe amblyopia is inappropriate. The confusion lies in the fact that amblyopia does not come from the lack of use of the eye, but has many causes that I shall explain. Amblyopia is the most common cause of visual loss in young children and therefore, it is important to understand it and to act immediately to try to correct it. In most cases, if recognized before the age of four, it can be treated and vision improved. Between the age of four and nine, there is less chançe to improve vision.

What can cause amblyopia? The most common cause is a misalignment of a child's eye from birth. When infants appear crossed at birth, they should be examined by an ophthalmologist who will determine if the infant has strabismus or pseudo (false) strabismus. Strabismus is the term used for eyes that cross in (Esotropia) or out (Exotropia). Some parents feel that their infant has a turned in eye. In actuality, the nasal skin fold, which is wider in infants, may cover the white part of the eye, giving the false appearance of an eye that is turned in. This condition is called pseudostrabismus. In order to confirm the presence or absence of strabismus, the eye physician uses a flashlight centered on both eyes to determine the position of the light on the cornea as the eye moves from right to left. She covers each eye individually and watches the movement of the eye behind the patch as it is covered and uncovered.

By the means of this technique she can determine if the eyes are aligned and appear to have their visual axis directed at the target. The physician notes the presence or absence of jerky eye movement (nystagmus) or evidence of restriction of the eyes as they move from right to left. The eye exam also includes a dilated exam to rule out a refractive problem and a retinal exam to evaluate the back of the eye and the media within the eye fully. "Media" is an ophthalmologist's term for the jelly within the eye. This jelly or gel maintains the volume of the eye. With the aid of an indirect ophthalmoscope, an instrument used with a handheld lens for looking in the back of the eye, she can also note the presence or absence of congenital cataracts which can block light from entering the newborn infant's eye.

As previously noted, the macula or visual center is poorly developed at birth. It needs light to enter the eye unimpeded in order to mature normally as the infant grows. If a blockage exists, either due to a congenital cataract or retinal abnormalities, vision will be decreased or absent. Visual deficit or loss will lead to misalignment of the eye. This condition was once termed deprivation amblyopia. This is easy to understand because light has been deprived from entering the eye by the existence of a blockage. Infants three months of age or younger fall into the category of being prone to develop this type of amblyopia. If light has difficulty entering the eyes, as in the case of congenital cataracts.

Other conditions may also decrease the amount of light entering an infant's eye. These are:

1. Malformation of the eyelids, causing a small opening between the upper and lower lids and an inability to lift the lid, commonly known as droopy eye lid. The term physicians use is *ptosis*. Infants do not outgrow this condition. An eye physician must assess the child's visual potential in these cases. If the eye's pupil is spared and not blocked, vision is usually good. If the pupil is covered, the physician can attempt to tape the infant's upper lid with non-allergenic tape during the day in order to allow light to penetrate the eye. I wish to stress that when we check the eye for the complaint at hand we always examine the entire eye.

2. A cloudy cornea or an opaque cornea termed a *leukoma* may be present. This finding may also decrease the amount of light entering the infant's eye.

Although the above are not often seen, they may occur without a previous family history of these conditions. They may also occur without a history of difficulty at birth. Low birth weight has been implicated as a high risk factor in strabismus and in myopia or nearsightedness. There are many types of strabismus, commonly referred to as cross eyes or an eye turn. I shall discuss the most common types that present themselves to our office.

Esotropia-In this condition the eyes may be turned in at birth. A parent might notice one eye or both eyes turning in alternatively. The pediatrician my caution the parent to defer an eye exam. The parent might be told that the infant might outgrow the problem, especially if there is no family history of it. If the symptoms do not disappear by six months of age, an eye exam is necessary. Babies who consistently favor one eye while they turn the other eye in toward the nose could develop Amblyopia in the turned in, weaker eye. Eyes that alternate have a better chance of equal vision, in other words, a better prognosis for good vision. Many believe esotropia is due to neurogenic influences. At times, fibrous bands like straps present at birth attach to the eye muscles resulting in loss of normal muscle function.

Esotropia can also be inherited. This fact should be disclosed to the pediatrician when providing a history. We have discussed eyes that turn at birth, a condition that contributes to loss of vision if not recognized by the parent or the pediatrician. The child should be referred to an eye physician in order to rule out other factors which could contribute to the eye turn. Refractive problems other than congenital factors can cause vision to be decreased and subsequently result in loss of fixation and an eye turn.

The following refractive conditions fall into the category of potentially decreasing vision if not corrected:

High on the list is unilateral high astigmatism, and high hyperopia, or farsightedness, either in one eye or both. High hyperopia or excessive farsightedness means that the infant needs to expend more effort to focus and see clearly up close as he accommodates. This triggers a neurologic mechanism, pulling the eyes in or converging. As they converge the eyes may overshoot, thereby creating a visible turn. If refractive problems are the only source of the eyes turning in, glasses, plus patching, if necessary, will correct the problem effectively and useful vision can be restored with time.

The road to vision is not always smooth and parents must be determined to follow the doctor's directions in order to succeed; working together as a team on behalf of the child is essential. After determining the stronger or dominant eye, the doctor will ask the parent to place a special patch which the doctor will provide, over the dominant eye, the eye that is usually or always straight. The decision to patch an eye is based on the need to restore vision in the amblyopic or weaker eye. In instances where there is little difference between vision of the two eyes, the doctor might elect to follow the patient closely and defer patching. The length of time that a patient wears a patch usually depends on his age – one half hour each day for a six month old patient and one hour per day for older children up to three years of age.

Patching is not always constant. Patching schedules may be altered or even eliminated once visual improvement occurs. A recognizable turn can totally disappear once visual stability is restored. I have never felt that total occlusion or wearing a patch over one eye was an effective approach for small children. Small children have labile vision. The visual strength of the eye under the patch can be lost resulting in that eye becoming amblyopic. This condition is called *occlusion amblyopia.* Once a child is asked to wear a patch the parent must be diligent in keeping follow-up appointments. If asked to plan special tasks with their child, such as asking her to perform near activities, i.e., reading, dot to dot, tracing, cut outs, pasting, Lego, and watching television during the patching time, the parent must stay with the child during the course of the activity.

There is only a small window of opportunity to restore vision with patching. This technique is not considered successful after the age of nine. Because patching is a difficult task for both children as well as their parents, it is important that amblyopia is detected at the earliest age possible. It is easier for the parent to begin patching before school starts and it is easier to handle the child's lack of compliance at the preschool age. Once the child enters kindergarten peer pressure can present a problem. The most difficult eye problems occur when one eye suffers severe vision loss or deep amblyopia. Restoration of vision in such a case cannot always be achieved. The child often rebels by removing the patch, even with a bribe, or looking over and under glasses.

As previously stated, if parents maintain a firm resolve, the reward is great. If the patient is in preschool, it is important to enlist the teacher's assistance to ensure that the patching schedule is carried out. If the child needs to wear her glasses constantly, the teacher should report any difficulties that may arise while she is wearing them. Some physicians use drops to blur vision in the preferred eye, thereby avoiding patches. I have never liked this approach because of the possible side effects of these drugs and the difficulty of reversing the action of the drug, namely prolonged dilation. In addition, these children tend to complain of problems with light sensitivity or photophobia because their pupil is essentially paralyzed for a time and they cannot use the eye for close up activities such as reading. Reversing the action of the drug even when deemed necessary is not always immediate. The doctor has better control with patching and greater success with that treatment, especially in a compliant patient with a dedicated parent.

As part of the discussion with parents regarding their child's prognosis and course of treatment, I have emphasized the importance of having the use of both eyes, in other words, achieving binocularity. Without binocularity many skills that we take for granted are lost to us. This means not having normal stereopsis. Children who are mainly monocular cannot compete in such sports as baseball, basketball, tennis, archery, etc. and should be encouraged to pursue sports that do not require good stereopsis, such as swimming, rowing, running, and wrestling. In addition, loss of an eye affects the child's choice of a future career or occupation, i.e., a pilot or surgeon. An irate parent called to tell me that her son could not join the air force because he wanted to become a pilot and he flunked the depth perception test. Unfortunately, this mother had stopped patching before her son's vision was fully restored.

2- *Exotropia*-is another eye turn we commonly see in an ophthalmic practice. In this condition the eye or eyes turn out. At times, one eye always appears divergent or turned out. This eye never returns to the straight or primary position. At times the eyes will alternate and a parent will say that they both turn out. The question is always asked, 'Does he seem to favor one eye?' During the eye exam the physician will determine if the turn is present only while the patient gazes at a distant object or if it is present when he gazes at a near point, such as in reading. The latter condition is called *convergence insufficiency*. This occurs if muscle weakness is noticeable as the child tries to read and he cannot hold his focus for a normal period of time before his eye drifts. In order to correct this problem the patient is instructed to perform special exercises which will strengthen his ability to maintain fixation at near long enough to read without getting tired. By practicing this exercise of fixing and holding eyes on the near object, fixation images of both eyes will fuse into one, creating a 3D effect.

There are some patients with the diagnosis of convergence insufficiency that actually have this muscle weakness and consequently are genuinely helped by doing prescribed exercises. However, we also find that use of muscle exercises in patients who do not have convergence insufficiency has gotten out of hand and misused by nonphysicians. These individuals falsely claim that children fail at reading because of poor muscle control and encourage parents to return frequently to their office for exercises. When examined in our office we find that these children have normal stereopsis. Reading actually only requires one good eye. Parents should be on their guard and seek another opinion from an eye physician when advised to have their children begin a series of weekly exercises.

Children who manifest an exotropia of a mechanical nature, not convergence insufficiency, may be a good candidate for surgical correction of the problem. This is especially true if they have good vision in both eyes. Parents have asked me if this is just cosmetic why should they place their child at risk to anesthesia and surgery? In the first instance correcting exotropia surgically is not for appearance alone. This type of surgery has a high success rate. Therefore, it could remove the stigma that children face when they grow into adulthood and friends and potential employers are looking at their eyes wondering which one is actually looking at them. However, the best reason to correct exotropia surgically, if the opportunity arises, is to regain some stereopsis. Following a good surgical result, and in the presence of good stable vision in both eyes, vision training can be implemented with an orthoptist. This is an individual who works with the eye physician in eye muscle training. Glasses may play a role in convergence insufficiency along with exercises. However, glasses alone are not successful in reducing a large outward deviation of the eye. If surgery is recommended, the operation can be delayed until the child is at least three years old. Since muscle surgery is done under general anesthesia, it is wise to wait and avoid the possibility of post operative morbidity. I have known surgeons who prefer to operate on babies after six months of age because they feel this provides a better chance to lock-in stereopsis. I disagree. You increase the anesthetic risk. It is also difficult to assess visual acuity perfectly at six months of age and until vision is equal in both eyes surgery is usually unsuccessful. The name of the game is VISION. That is what we strive for. First it is always necessary to build and secure good vision before considering any type of strabismus surgery.

The following are some tips to look for if you think your child might have a muscle problem not detected by others:

1. He has a funny head position and always favors one eye.
2. He keeps his head or chin up, or down.
3. He closes one eye when looking in the distance or up close.
4. He tilts his head.
5. He sometimes sees double.
6. Objects come and go.

If the doctor determines that the eye exam is negative for a muscle problem the following conditions could exist:

1. a compensatory mechanism
2. a habit that the child assumed in order to improve his visual acuity.
3. *ocular torticollis*, a condition associated with weak muscles in the back of the neck. These children are often referred to orthopedic physicians.

TYPES OF STRABISMUS

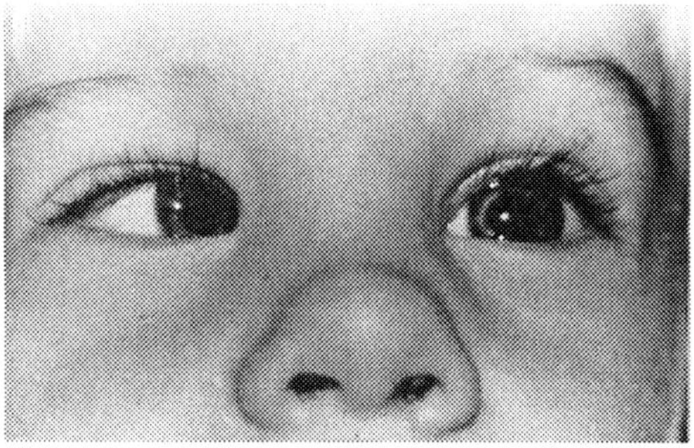

Figure 1
Esotropia

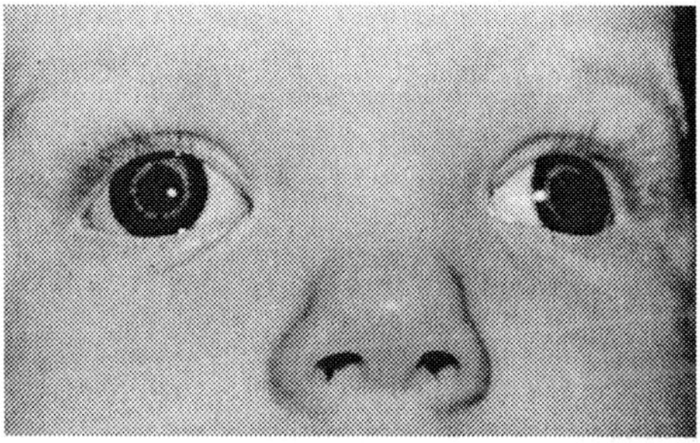

Figure 2
Exotropia

CHAPTER IV

NORMAL APPEARANCE OF NEWBORN'S EYES AND ORBITS AT BIRTH

1 – Most normal newborns have eyes that appear slightly turned out. This is termed *exodeviation*. The anatomic position of the eyes in the bony socket, the *orbit*, creates this appearance. By the age of six months the muscles that pull the eyes in have strengthened and the *exodeviation* should no longer exist. If the baby's eyes still continue to look turned out, she should be referred to an ophthalmologist.

2 – A newborn with a hemorrhage around the whites of the eye is not uncommon. If the mother had a difficult delivery there may be also retinal hemorrhages present. If this occurs, or is suspected, the neonate, or newborn, should be referred to an eye doctor upon discharge for evaluation. Generally, superficial redness on the surface of the neonate's eyes will slowly absorb without any subsequent visual damage.

3 – Redness and swelling localized to the upper lids is often due to prolonged or difficult births. This condition is called *fetal hyperemia*. As the infant matures, the appearance of the lids improve and redness disappears. No treatment is necessary and there is no cosmetic problem in later life.

4 – Normal tearing is usually present by the time an infant is three weeks of age. Absence of tears is rare and often associated with other findings. Should a parent be concerned if the neonate has a discharge from one or both eyes? Yes. It could mean the presence of an infection. If the newborn presents with thick, yellowish, or so called *mucoid* tears, the mother should have her vaginal secretions examined. It is not uncommon for neonates to develop an eye infection in the birth canal. If the discharge is visible at three days postpartum, a staph infection should be considered. The baby should be referred to an ophthalmologist who will examine the eyes and take an eye culture to determine the exact *etiology* of the disease. If any infection is present, antibiotics either in the form of eye ointments or systemic liquid antibiotics are prescribed. The parent is also instructed to wash the eye lids with cotton and warm water twice daily. In addition, I have instructed parents how to massage the area under the lid toward the nose. It is helpful to press gently over this area where the tear sac is located in order to express mucus which collects in the sac during an infection. If these infections are not treated properly they can cause a chronically irritated red eye, skin irritation or dermatitis, and even lead to a blocked tear duct. Tear duct obstruction is discussed in a separate chapter.

It has been established that the eye grows fastest in the first year of life, approximately 3. 8 mm in length and then continues to grow slowly until puberty. Fifty percent of the volume of the eye, the ocular diameter and surface area, is established by six months of age. [1] These facts explain why an infant's refraction changes continuously as she matures. Inherited factors, such as farsightedness or near-sightedness, will play a part in children's ultimate visual acuity and the possible need for glasses. Nearsighted children usually start wearing glasses between eight and nine years old.

Orbital spaces in which the eyes sit are called sockets. They are usually symmetrical. The shape could be compared to a quadrilateral pyramid. Children have small orbital spaces. Consequently, the eyes normally appear close together. As the eyes grow, the socket also changes shape. With the growth of the facial sinuses such as the *frontal* and *ethmoidal* sinuses the eyes are no longer as close together. In children, the *maxillary sinus*, the ones in the cheek area, are small. The frontal sinuses do not become well developed until after the age of nine. These are important facts to understand since the orbit and the tissues that surround it are affected by many conditions which will be discussed in later chapters.

---

[1] Isenberg, Sherwin, The Eye In Infancy, Year Book Medical Publishers, 1989.

CHAPTER V

THE ROLE OF THE PEDIATRICIAN IN DETECTING EYE PROBLEMS AT BIRTH

The following story serves to emphasize the importance of good history taking, careful observation and knowledge. Your pediatrician examines your newborn. The baby was full term. The delivery was uneventful without any problem in the delivery room. You notice that your baby appears to have a white pupil. There was no history of the use of forceps. Can babies be found to have eye problems even with a normal birth history? Yes. The pediatrician diagnoses a *leukoria*, a Greek term for a white pupil. She also tells you that this could be a congenital cataract. She tells you to be calm. The diagnosis cannot be accurate without a thorough exam by an ophthalmologist. She refers you without delay. While your baby is in the pediatrician's office, he is checked for hearing deficiency and skin lesions. You ask the doctor what to expect at the time of the eye examination and are told the following: as a parent you should have an eye exam before or after you baby's visit. The eye doctor will look in the back of your eye. The finding of retinal problems or a small congenital cataract could be helpful in determining the diagnosis in your baby's case. She will take a more detailed birth history, including your medical history. She looks for specific information which relates to eye problems. She will question you about such things as viral infections in the first trimester of pregnancy, exposure to measles, and having cats in your home. You will be asked to list any medications you took during your pregnancy. A family history of a relative with vision problems or eye surgery may be relevant.

The following is an account of what a parent can expect the ophthalmologist to do during the baby's eye examination. She measures the diameter of the shiny part of the eye. This part of the surface of the eye is called the cornea. This is simply done with a special ruler. The axial length of the eye can be determined with the use of ultrasound, a noninvasive test performed in the office without anesthesia. Infants tolerate the test very well. There is no pain associated with this very useful diagnostic tool. Before attempting an ultrasound on an infant, the mother aids the doctor by offering the baby a bottle or pacifier.

Even though the baby was referred to her office with the presumptive diagnosis of congenital cataract, the physician must search for other conditions which could cause a cataract. In order to rule out the presence of a tumor or a retinal detachment not clearly defined even with ultrasound, the parent is told that because of the seriousness of the problem, further testing must be performed under anesthesia. At this time, the eye doctor attempts to visualize the retinal surface and its contents. This is difficult because the cataract may completely obstruct the view. Valuable information can be gained if the light can penetrate through the dilated pupil. A hand held device called a tonometer takes the pressure of the eye. This information is necessary in order to rule out glaucoma, or shrinkage of the ocular contents and poor eye volume. If the back of the eye, the retina, that is often described as the film in a camera, cannot be visualized satisfactorily, the eye doctor orders an MRI, a magnetic resonance imaging scan. This test can rule out the most serious problems such as eye tumors. If after this thorough examination the only positive finding is a congenital cataract, the doctor might recommend surgery to remove the cataract.

When cataracts occur, the lens of the eye has become white or cloudy. If it completely blocks light from entering the back of the eye, the normal growth and development of the macula is impaired. As I previously discussed, the macula is essentially the most important area in the retina for fine acuity. Even after a successful cataract extraction, prognosis for functional vision is often guarded. I have always felt that vision is precious. Parents should be guided by their eye surgeon if their infant is in good medical health. The modern techniques used by today's eye surgeons have resulted in good visual outcomes. Again I advocate parents to be sensitive observers of possible eye problems in their infants and not to delay in determining the true condition of their children's eyes.

We have discussed congenital cataracts without other ocular findings and what prognosis these infants face. What if there are other physical findings associated with infantile cataracts, such as a peculiar shaking or back and forth movement of the eyes. You describe this to the eye doctor as not smooth movement but more like a pendulum. She tells you that this is called *nystagmus*. In addition, she goes on to state that the presence of *nystagmus* in an infant with a congenital cataract can be a sign of decreased visual acuity. If your infant has cataract in both eyes or bilaterally, the most dense cataract is usually operated on first.

While the infant is under anesthesia, the surgeon attempts to determine the refractive power of the eyes, i.e., very nearsighted or very farsighted. This information is necessary in order to determine the need for an implant at a later date or corrective lenses. Adults receive intraocular implants following cataract surgery. Children, however, have to be individually evaluated. The surgeon may not elect to implant a lens initially because of the following factors:

1. The child is too young.
2. The lens would have to remain in the eye too long
3. The growth of the eye might create power changes which dramatically alter the original calculation.

It is better to be conservative and delay implantation to a later date. Vision restoration can be achieved with the aid of contacts or glasses during the waiting period. It is true that implant surgery provides the eye with greater optical resolution and stability of vision. Therefore, when appropriate, the goal is to implant a lens into the child's eye.

During the period of visual rehabilitation following cataract surgery patching the good eye, the non-amblyopic eye, is necessary. The parent receives a patching schedule and appointments for follow up. After the operation, the eye is termed aphakic, without a lens. Glasses or contacts are prescribed as a temporary solution. If the child can be fitted with contacts and the parent will cooperate, contact lenses are more effective in providing for a better resolution of the difference in image size between the aphakic eye and the eye that still has its natural lens. The brain cannot fuse a difference of greater than

30 percent of one eye over the other. Even with a successful contact lens wearer there is often a residual image difference. If children had binocularity prior to the onset of cataracts, wearing contacts following surgery will provide them with a better chance to reestablish binocularity. Children without binocularity and greater visual deficits prior to surgery may subsequently only regain peripheral fusion. To have even a little fusion is important because it enhances the stability of the eye thereby helping to maintain better alignment. As previously mentioned some of these children also have strabismus or muscle problems. Cataract surgery is often an uphill battle but with early detection and the advent of new scientific methods successful visual restoration has become a greater possibility.

There are other conditions that your pediatrician might discover when she exams your infant at birth. The baby appears to have hazy looking eyes, or cloudy corneas. Some corneal edema or haze which occurs shortly after birth will clear spontaneously. Those that represent serious congenital problems such as congenital glaucoma must be ruled out. Therefore it is best to be referred to an ophthalmologist if a cloudy cornea is suspected. The physician will also ask the parent questions regarding possible infections, i.e., herpes, rubella and syphilis, during pregnancy which could cause intrauterine inflammation of the cornea in the newborn. A history of forceps delivery is noteworthy since this can cause trauma to a baby's cornea as well as a *periocular subconjunctival hemorrhage,* a condition in which the whites of the eye are red at birth. The pediatrician checks for the presence or absence of skin *hemangioma*, a vascular skin lesion called

Sturge-Weber, in and around the eyelid and face. Congenital glaucoma can be associated with Sturge-Weber when the so called port wine stain involves the upper lid. As discussed earlier, if there are any potential problems that can not easily be explained the baby must be referred to an ophthalmologist.

During the eye exam the parent is asked whether she noticed if her baby showed signs of light sensitivity or increased tearing. These symptoms can be present in association with a cloudy cornea in congenital glaucoma. Although this disease is extremely rare, it is noteworthy to mention because failure to detect its early signs can lead to blindness. The eye physician measures the size of the cornea. A cloudy cornea that is larger than the average size in diameter and associated with tearing is strongly suggestive of congenital glaucoma. The parent is told that the baby needs to be examined under anesthesia in order to complete the examination. The following steps are planned: 1- the intraocular pressure is taken; 2-the front of the eye, i.e., the cornea, anterior chamber, the angle of the eye and the lens, are examined under the surgical microscope; and 3- the back of the eye is viewed to determine the health of the optic nerve and the retina.

Science has provided us with diagnostic and surgical tools which enable us to have successful visual outcomes but we as parents must have a greater understanding of the eye and the presenting symptoms that may or may not lead to their infant's loss of vision.

Another common finding that an otherwise normal baby can have at birth is a *dermoid*, a benign tumor that appears as either a partial or total white opacification or appear as a lump in the upper lid. At times this congenital tumor can be large enough to obstruct the visual axis and thereby decrease the visual potential of the eye. It is round, contains hair and sweat glands. It is pinkish gray in color. If present it is important to recognize since many of these infants have other developmental problems. The doctor should test for corneal desensitization in cases of opaque cornea. Lack of corneal sensitivity can lead to opaque corneas. The test is simply done with a cotton swab lightly brushed across the surface of the cornea. A positive result is recorded when the infant blinks. If the view in is diminished by the corneal opacity, ultrasound can be used to validate the health of the eye.

DERMOID CYST

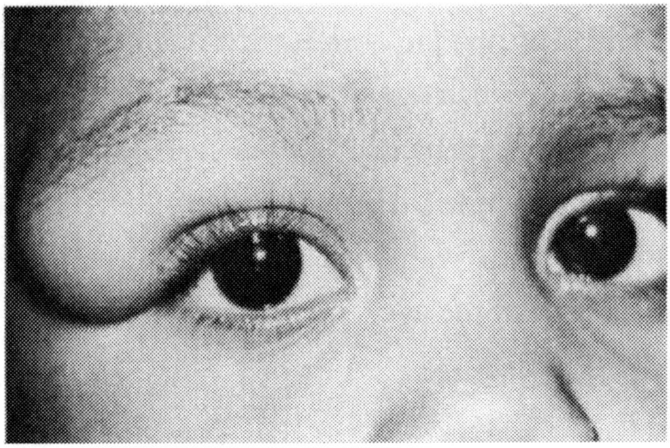

Typical Location

CHAPTER VI

CONJUNCTIVITIS OR THE "RED EYE" IN THE NEWBORN

Conjunctivitis, erroneously called *pink eye*, can be present in many normal neonates following delivery and is very common. It can lead to chronic tearing problems if not treated properly at its inception. It is wrong to call red eyes with chronic discharge *pink eye*. Pink is a color. There are many organisms that can cause redness in a baby's eyes. Originally pink eye was attributed to a virus. In newborns, conjunctivitis was found to be caused primarily by bacteria. When asked to describe the discharge on the lids and skin around the infants eyes, the parent states that the discharge can start like mucus and change in color with the length of time of the infection. This is so because the color of the discharge changes with the severity of the infection. In addition, the lids can be swollen and crusty. The discharge is irritating to the skin around the eyelids and should be gently removed with warm water and cotton.

Parents should record the day the discharge started. If the symptoms presented within 48 hours of birth, the cause may be attributed to preventive measures to reduce infection either with silver nitrate swabs or mild antibiotic drops used in the nursery. These preventive measures have been known to cause allergic reactions in some newborns. Other infections which present from 2-5 days following birth may be from the mother's birth canal. If the onset of redness and discharge starts around the fourth day to one week after birth, staph infection is the most likely cause. Another agent which can cause conjunctivitis after 1-4 weeks postpartum and is more difficult to treat is chlamydia. In order to determine which organism is involved, the ophthalmologist uses a cotton swab to collect the secretion from the inside of the baby's eyelid. A culture tube is sent to the lab. Once the organism has been identified, specific antibiotics are prescribed. In addition, parents are told to wash the baby's eyelids daily with cotton and warm water. They are also instructed to massage the area close to the nose under the lid called the tear sac. This sac can hold bacteria and be filled with secretions which contribute to chronic infection.

History has shown that in our attempt to protect the newborn from post partum infection we have found ourselves facing a quandary as to what prophylaxis is best in the nursery. In some states prophylaxis is required by law. As early as 1880, silver nitrate has been used as prophylaxis. Although effective against gonorrhea as well as staph aureus and e. coli, it has not been proven useful fighting cases of Chlamydia. The use of 0.5 percent erythromycin ointment is more effective against Chlamydia. It is now used as an agent in many nurseries. Erythromycin ointment is also less irritating to the lining of the newborns' eyes. Consequently it will not cause chemical conjunctivitis or *pink eye*. Prophylaxis against eye infection is even provided to infants delivered by caesarean section.

CHAPTER VII

INFECTIOUS DISEASES A SPECIFIC FORM OF CONJUNCTIVITIS OR RED EYE

This subject was touched upon in Chapter VI "Conjunctivitis or the "RED EYE". Infectious disease of the eye is a common problem. It can cause serious risks to vision especially in newborns or following ocular trauma.

In this section I shall discuss how eye infections are acquired at birth. Since the inception of prophylaxis against infection, the incidence of newborn eye infections as well as conjunctivitis of delayed onset at 1-21 days has been dramatically reduced. Despite great strides in protecting the newborn infant from serious eye contamination, the fact of life is that venereal disease is still part of our medical scene and must be considered when neonates get conjunctivitis postnatally around day four. Parents usually do not notice the red eye with the creamy discharge until day six, when the baby is already home. The eyelids are markedly swollen and the lids are stuck together. An immediate eye exam is necessary since this is a very contagious eye infection. This type of conjunctivitis is treatable once the bacteria has been identified with the aid of a culture. If left untreated, damage to the cornea could result. Fortunately, this type of venereal disease is not as prevalent today. Other sexually transmitted infectious diseases have taken the place of syphilis and gonorrhea. Currently, Chlamydia is an organism which is also sexually transmitted. It has become more and more frequent as an agent of newborn conjunctivitis. It is the leading cause of non-gonorrheal urethritis in males and can be found to infect the female genitalia including the cervix. If neonates are exposed to Chlamydia at birth 74%[2] will develop conjunctivitis. Even newborns born by caesarean section can be exposed to Chlamydia especially with a history of ruptured membranes. Signs of infection usually occur from 4-12 days after birth. The infant's eyes are mildly red. The lids are swollen and on examination the lining of the lower lids are bumpy, not smooth.

Herpes Simplex, as previously mentioned, can affect the lids. It can be found in the conjuntiva of neonates as well as in adults. Both age groups can present with similar findings. These findings include lid swelling, a red lid lining and what the eye doctor considers a telltale cloudy cornea or surface of the eye. A special dye test called flourescein is used to detect a pattern that is specific for herpes involvement in the cornea. Unfortunately, when herpes is found in a neonate, other areas of infection may be present throughout the body and should be evaluated.

Common bacterial infections have been cultured from the eyes of newborns. The most often seen are Staphylococcus, Streptococcus, and even E. Coli. As previously mentioned, as early as 1880, prophylaxis was initiated

---

[2] Isenberg, Sherwin, The Eye In Infancy; Year Book Medical Publishers, 1989

against these infections with the aid of silver nitrate. Most states now require that all newborns receive a form of prophylaxis. Unfortunately, silver nitrate has been found to be caustic to the lining of the eye in some cases. Causing a condition referred to as chemical conjunctivitis. If redness is due to silver nitrate it will disappear without treatment in a few days. If the baby develops a discharge in and around the eye which persists longer than three days the parent should suspect a bacterial infection.

If a newborn has had a red eye while in the nursery, upon discharge, a referral should be made to an eye doctor's office in order to rule out late onset conjunctivitis. This is because silver nitrate has not proven to be enough prophylaxis against many newborn eye infections. Currently both silver nitrate and antibiotic ointments such as .5% erythromycin ointment or 1% tetracycline ointment are used in different institutions. Both the Centers for Disease Control and the American Academy of Pediatrics have established guidelines for the use of these ointments. Cases of sexually transmitted infectious diseases causing eye infections in newborns require the administration of systemic antibiotics. In these cases, it is recommended that both the pediatrician and the ophthalmologist be in attendance.

CHAPTER VIII

TEARING

Tearing in a newborn who does not have conjunctivitis is not uncommon, but is it normal and what does it indicate? How long should a parent wait before addressing the issue? Babies usually start producing tears around three months of age. If this does not happen, parents should inform their pediatrician. The eye needs a normal amount of tears to protect the cornea and clear debris from getting into it. Without sufficient tears the cornea dries and erosions occur.

There is an enzyme found in tears which has antibacterial properties protecting the eye from infections. During emotional moments or when the eye is irritated, tears from the tear gland or *lacrimal gland* flow spontaneously. There are also accessory glands which add to the tear secretion. The drainage system is comprised of a opening called a *punctum,* or hole, which leads into a conduit or *nasolacrimal duct*. This duct goes into the nasal passage. A membrane, essentially a valve in the nasal mucosa or lining, opens to allow the tears to enter the nose, usually at birth. If the membrane between the duct and the nasal mucosa persists, nasolacrimal duct obstruction occurs. With proper medical treatment, i.e., erythromycin ointment and massaging of the tear sac, the nasolacrimal duct will be open in most cases by six months of age. If after this time your infant is still bothered by crusting of the lids and tearing, visit your ophthalmologist. She will determine if the tear duct problem is the result of chronic infection or a mechanical obstruction. If after a culture is taken and antibiotic treatment specific for the bacteria found in the eye fails to resolve the problem, she may decide to probe the tear duct. The procedure is done under light anesthesia in order to have the infant's full cooperation. Many physicians encourage parents to bring their infants in for probing as soon as the excess tearing begins. I always favored antibiotics, massaging the sac and following up for possible conjunctivitis. This method of treatment cured most of my patients; only the refractory infants needed to have probing. When contemplating general anesthesia in an infant it is always safer to give them time to mature, in other words, wait as along as medically feasible.

CHAPTER IX

TEAR DUCT OBSTRUCTION

This subject needs special mention. This condition is found in 6%[3] of normal newborns. It causes excessive tearing and secondary infection in the eye with the blocked tear duct. At times both eyes can be affected. The obstruction clears spontaneously in most cases by the time the infant is six months to one year old. As mentioned, the obstruction is due to the persistence of a membrane inside the turbinate of the nose which blocks the tears from flowing into the nose along a normal path. The tears back up into the eye and pool under the lower lid mixing with mucus. During the time when infants are bothered by excessive tearing and redness in and around the eye it is best to follow a simple routine. Parents should wash the baby's lids with cotton and warm water to remove crusts that form on the skin, thus preventing skin irritation. Massage the area of the tear sac gently as instructed by their physician. She will take a culture of the discharge seen on the lashes and in the eye in order to determine the need for antibiotic therapy. If tearing persists despite treatment with massages and antibiotics, the final step is nasolacrimal probing under general anesthesia. Since even light general anesthesia poses some risk to babies, it is

---

[3] Isenberg, Sherwin; The Eye In Infancy; Year Book Medical Publishers, 1989

important that their pediatrician clears them for surgery. The eye doctor would advocate probing the tear duct only in severe protracted cases and not because a parent is impatient or annoyed with a persistent condition.

Tearing is a symptom. It is not only found in children with blocked tear ducts but can also be seen in silver nitrate reactions, viral eye conditions and in congenital glaucoma. An ophthalmologist needs to evaluate a tearing problem in order to determine its cause. Tears are very important to the eye. They act as a protective mantel and help fight infection. The eye gets its moisture from glands in the lining of the lids. The primary source of tears is from the tear gland or *lacrimal gland.* The eye will tear when it is touched or when it experiences irritation. This is not the normal tear flow that bathes the eye but is a reactive tearing or so called reflex tearing. Absence of reflex tearing is very rare and can cause serious vision problems.

TEAR DUCT OBSTRUCTION

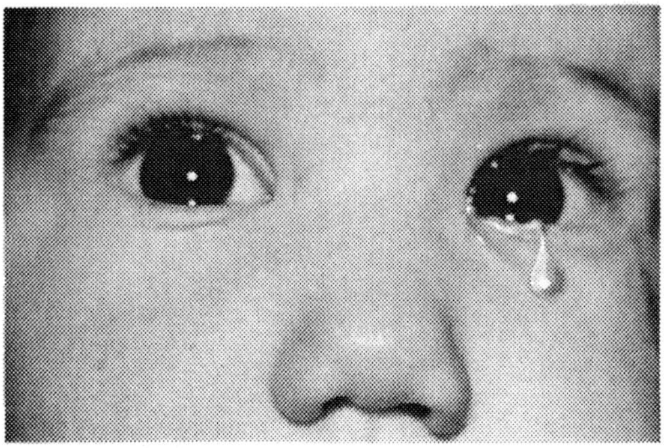

A "wet look" to lashes

CHAPTER X

DROOPY LID OR PTOSIS

I have discussed many eye problems that normal infants can present with at birth. One of the most distressing to parents is called a droopy eyelid, or *ptosis*. Physicians often use the word *blepharoptosis* in their discussion of "droopy eyelids." This is because the blephara are the lids and ptosis refers to the relaxation of the eyelids. This condition can affect one or both eyes. Even though we search for a congenital origin, often there is none. Many cases of ptosis are caused by ocular muscles that are weak and underdeveloped. Ptosis is often associated with widening of the skin on either side of the nose. This area is called the *epicanthus*. In this case a shortage of skin contracts the fold thereby changing the eye opening or aperture.

Pictured are types of epicanthi problems;

LID AND EPICANTHAL PROBLEMS

1-(Figure 1) The eyelids are mildly lowered but the pupil is spared and there is no loss of vision. The skin fold, or epicanthus, extends from the lower lid upward into the upper lid.

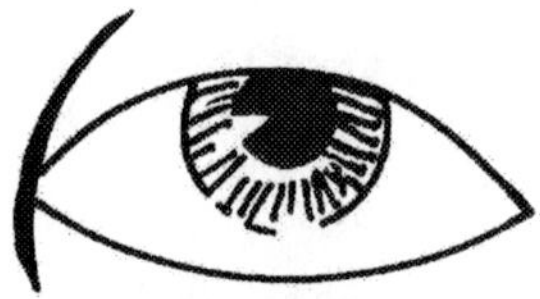

Figure 1
Lowered Lid Pupil Spared

2-(Figure 2) The skin fold can be wide in infants, at times giving the false appearance that the eye is turned in when it is not. This is called *pseudostrabismus*. As the child matures, the condition usually disappears.

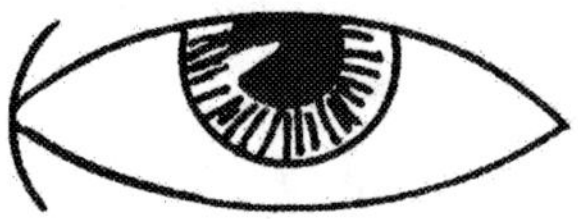

Figure 2
Wide Skin Fold- Pseudostrabismus

3-(Figure 3) The upper and lower lids are tight and the eyes appear "slit-like". There is a missing lid fold and loss of ability to elevate the eye. Surgical correction by an eye plastic surgeon can be effective.

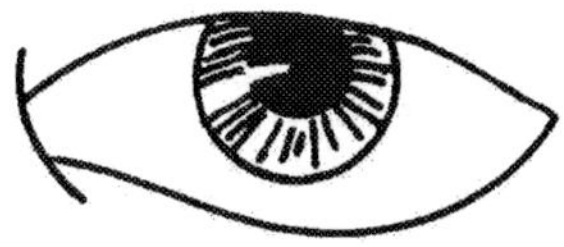

Figure 3
Tight Lids and Slit Like Appearance

PTOSIS OR DROOPY EYE

4-(Figure 4) This patient is unable to lift her right eye lid when she looks upwards. A congenital muscle problem is most often the cause. Surgical correction is necessary for cosmetic reasons and to prevent loss of vision or amblyopia. Note a downward position of the eyelashes can occur, which as discussed could cause corneal problems.

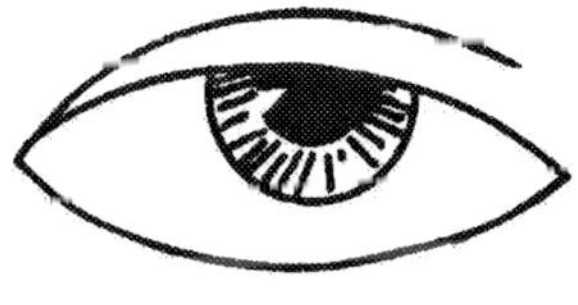

Figure 4

Droopy Eye Lid secondary
to lack of muscle function

If the eye is normal, and the lid does not cover the pupil, vision should not be affected and amblyopia will not occur. However astigmatism could result from the upper lid pressing on the cornea over a period of time during the maturation of the child's eye. The configuration of the lids can contribute to recurrent eye infections. In addition, the eyelashes scratch the cornea because they can point downwards. The cornea should be tested to confirm the presence of a positive reflex or *Bell's Phenomenon*. Regular follow-up visits are necessary to prevent loss of vision if there is lid alteration as the child grows. Eye plastic surgeons specializing in ptosis correction may wait until the infant matures. The timing for this surgical correction depends on the severity of the case and whether the patient could have loss of vision or amblyopia.

CHAPTER XI

EYELID PROBLEMS

Normal newborns can also have discoloration of their eyelids. The most common cause is blood or *hemangiomatous tumors*. They can appear like small flat strawberry marks, extensive enough to cover the upper lid. Benign strawberry-like tumors that are visible at birth or thereafter usually regress by seven years of age. A cat scan is recommended in order to determine the extension of the hemangioma in the lid and the orbit. The infant should be carefully monitored. No treatment is necessary unless vision is threatened by the presence of the lesion or bump. Astigmatism and subsequently amblyopia can result if the lid is heavily involved with the hemangioma. Parents should be prudent and cautious. They should not be anxious to correct the problem solely for cosmetic reasons. They should rely on the advice of those eye surgeons trained to handle vascular lesions in and around the eyes. Laser surgery has proven effective in treating some types of hemangiomas.

The most common nonmalignant eyelid bump seen in infants and children is called a *chalazion*. A chalazion results from an obstruction of a duct in a gland, a *meibomian gland*. It can start as a smooth red bump on the inside of the upper or lower lid. It can extend to the lid margin and appear to have a white head. The chalazion can easily spread throughout the entire lid creating a hot swollen purulent, or pussy, lid. Inflammation of the base of the eyelashes can predispose the child to chalazia. It has also been said that eye strain and improper glasses contribute to the formation of chalazia. Your eye physician will take a culture of the discharge to determine the organism involved, prescribe antibiotics, eye ointment, warm soaks and eyelid scrubs. If the problem does not resolve itself with maximum medication over a period of time, the chalazion can be surgically excised. Unfortunately local anesthesia is necessary. Eye physicians elect to use general anesthesia more often with infants and children than adults because the former become too agitated.

There are other growths of a noninfectious nature that can appear spontaneously on the eyelids of children. They are benign skin tags or warts, sometimes referred to as *papillomas*. If they are annoying or cosmetically unattractive they can simply be excised without significant pain or cosmetic disfigurement.

I have discussed *dermoids* in the section regarding corneal opacity. They can more commonly present under or in the upper lid on the temporal side. The parent will notice a smooth bulge and discoloration when the infant cries. This embryonic growth or dermoid is not malignant. It is firm to the touch and not painful, but is does not respond to ointments or antibiotics, The dermoid can be easily excised under general anesthesia. Parents should wait until the child is old enough in order not to pose an anesthetic risk. Cosmetic appearance is excellent following excision.

Cellulitis, inflammation of the skin and muscle of the eye lid and abscess, are more serious problems that can occur and require immediate action. This condition is associated with swollen lymph glands located in front of the ear and under the jaw. The infection can start simply from a break in the skin due to an insect bite or penetrating injury, i.e., a stick or sharp toy. The child can have a high temperature and appear toxic or acutely sick. The nasal sinuses need to be evaluated to rule out the spread of infection to the ethmoid (near the nose) and maxillary sinuses (in the cheek area). The patient with positive findings of sinus involvement needs to have an Ear, Nose and Throat physician, as well as an eye doctor providing treatment and course of action. These children are usually hospitalized since they need systemic antibiotics and often surgical intervention consisting of incision and drainage in order to locate the abscess. In serious cases, the lids that are inflamed and puffy can be so prominent that the eye appears "popped out".

Bacterial skin infections can also affect the eyelids of infants and children. They may be due to a staph infection localized in a hair follicle (root) or a gland of the lid. It starts as a red area (stye) externally which grows wider and comes to a head as a pimple. Saline soaks are useful, followed by antibiotics which your eye physician will recommend based on bacterial sensitivity. Stye cream, often prescribed by pharmacists, is not helpful in this condition. *Impetigo,* a staph infection of the skin, can also present as pustules on the face and lids.

Viruses can also cause infections of the eyelids in children. The following are not uncommon:

1. Chicken Pox

2. Herpes Simplex (appears as fever blisters with clear fluid)

3. Molluscum (a small bump usually near the lid margin containing a depression in the center) These can cause conjunctivitis or inflammation of the skin around the eye.

4. Herpes Zoster, known as Shingles, can also affect the eyelids of small children. The virus causes a rash on the forehead and upper lid. It can be associated with neuralgic pain.

Noninfectious conditions that patients can present with are:

1. Louse infections of the scalp (Pediculosis or Nits) which are attached to the eyebrows and lashes. These nits have to be individually removed by the eye doctor at the slit lamp. These insects cause itching and redness of skin of the eyelid.

2. Poison Ivy can cause redness, swelling and blisters of the eyelids. This type of contact dermatitis can also be found when children are exposed to poison oak, sumac, ragweed, and cosmetics or ir-

ritants, such as some soaps or detergents. The physician must take a thorough history in order to remove the causative agent. I have found the use of local and/or systemic steroids to be helpful, as well as Benedryl in these cases.

SEVERE LID INFECTION

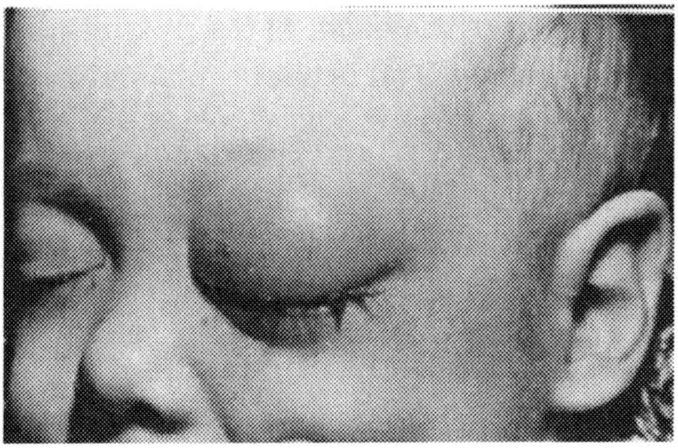

CELLULITIS

CHAPTER XII

EYE TRAUMA

We have all felt helpless when an infant or child cries out in pain. Injuries that occur in and around the eyes threaten vision and must be dealt with immediately. It has been said that half of all blindness is preventable. If this is true, it is a shocking revelation to learn that we are not making greater efforts to guard against possible eye injuries. In addition, as eye physicians, we also find that most vision loss occurs in the first decade of life. While all injuries cannot always be prevented, we can take steps to help avoid sports related injuries. Years ago I was a panelist for the National Society for The Prevention of Blindness in Children. The panel developed guidelines for eye protection which should be helpful to parents, teachers and coaches. For example, children should wear protective gear in all racquetball sports. Contact sports, i.e., football and wrestling, should not be encouraged in very near sighted children. Children who are highly myopic are at a greater risk if they participate in platform or springboard diving because the severe impact that occurs when they enter the water can cause tears in the retina. Boxing is notoriously unsafe in these children for the same reason. If your child wears glasses and you are not sure if the sport she has chosen is safe for her eyes, you should consult your ophthalmologist.

Head injuries which do not require hospitalization and do not seem serious to the pediatrician can still cause an ocular problem down the road. Holes and tears in the retina behind the eye can develop slowly with multiple impacts. A retinal detachment can occur much later in life. To avoid this unfortunate occurrence, the parent should inform the eye doctor of any instances of head injury.

Common Eye Injuries and How to Handle Them Efficiently and With Understanding

1- The parent should try to be calm and help her child be less anxious and more accommodating. Your child was playing in a sandbox, suddenly cries and rubs her eyes. This behavior should alert you to a foreign body entering and lodging under the lid. You should wash the injured eye with cotton and warm water. It is best to have a bottle of *sterile* eye irrigating solution in the medicine cabinet at all times, so that you can try to irrigate the eye gently. Look for hemorrhage around the eye and call your eye doctor. It is important to understand why an eye exam is necessary. A foreign body can cause damage to the child's cornea. The corneal abrasion that often results can be extremely painful. Sand can contain iron particles in it, which if allowed to remain in the eye can cause a rust ring. Your eye physician will remove this ring with the use of "feel better" topical anesthetic drops and a hand held instrument. This procedure is performed at the slit lamp. The cornea usually recovers its clarity.

2- Your child fell into bushes, or a playmate poked him in the eye with a stick, or something flew into his eye. You notice a black thing on the white of his eye. After irrigating the eye with *sterile* eye solution the foreign body does not move. Your child is crying in pain. Do not cover the eye with a patch but call your eye physician. Be prepared to give a complete history over the phone in order for her to decide if she needs to meet you in the emergency room or in the office. At times, even though you can see the foreign body, other material, wood or plant fragments, might lodge under the upper lid. The movement of the lid as the eye is opened and closed can cause linear abrasions to form on the corneal surface. The eye doctor can evaluate the corneal problem after seating your child behind the slit lamp (biomicroscope). She uses a special fluorescein dye which aids in detecting the depth and extent of the corneal abrasion. Antibiotics in the form of ointment and/or drops are placed in the eye. A patch may be placed on the eye depending on the size of the abrasion. Follow up appointments are always recommended.

3- Black eyes are not uncommon. They do not occur spontaneously in children as in the case of mature adults. Black eyes frequently occur from a punch in the eye, a toy thrown in the eye, an elbow, a fall, a head injury, a fall off a bicycle or a swing, an insect bite, or an insect flying into the eye, a finger in the eye, a contusion injury to other parts of the face, a tennis ball, racket ball to the orbital area, a fall down a flight of stairs and frequently falls from a high chair. We realize from this partial list of unfortunate possibilities that bringing up children can sometimes prove hazardous to their eyes. They challenge us to always be alert and respond quickly to signs of possible danger.

The following discussion will explain how to recognize probable problems and enable you to understand what might happen to the eye if they are present:

1- The eyelids are swollen, bluish or red. This is called lid *ecchymosis*. Apply a cold compress but do not wait until the lid improves. Call your eye physician and be prepared to provide a complete history. She will then be able to rule out the possibility of a so called blow out fracture of the bony area around the eye. She examines the eye for the presence of blood in the eye, or *hyphema*, the movement or lack of movement of the iris and pupil, pupil symmetry of one eye to the other, and pupillary reaction to light. She looks at the lens of the eye to rule out dislocation and traumatic cataract. The back of the eye is examined with an indirect ophthalmoscope through a dilated pupil. The retina is checked for the presence or absence of signs of trauma such as edema or swelling, folds in the retina, hemorrhage, contusion and even retinal detachment. A child might have pathology in his eyes even in the presence of good visual acuity. He does not complain of changes in his vision, but of pain on opening and closing his eyes because of the swelling and possible corneal abrasion. Even with almost closed eyelids, your doctor can in most cases diagnose the condition and treat the eye effectively. Treatment will depend on the type of injury sustained.

2- A foreign body or penetrating injury is suspected. Your child was poked in the eye with a stick or the point of a pen or knife. During the eye exam the following usually takes place: the eye is cleansed, topical anesthetic is instilled in it. The child sits behind the examining microscope, called a slit lamp. If there is a laceration in the eye, gentle probing can be performed to determine the depth of the laceration and if a foreign body is embedded in it. Superficial lacerations of the skin around the eye or conjunctiva do not usually require suturing since they heal well on their own.

If your child has been in a car accident and the examination in the emergency room was negative for an eye problem yet you continue to see a recurrent redness around the shiny part of the eye, this could be caused by a foreign body such as glass in the eye. Glass, once it penetrates the eye is not necessarily painful. It can lie dormant in the anterior space in front of the iris, acting as an irritant, thereby causing redness. A three year old child was seen in my office with a history of chronic redness of his right eye. The history included a car accident when he was a toddler. With the use of a special lens while seated at the slit lamp, I discovered the presence of a small fragment of glass lodged in the space of the eye in front of the iris called the *anterior chamber*. The glass was surgically removed and the redness disappeared.

The reader can now appreciate the fact that trauma to the eye must always be taken seriously. Careful evaluation of the ocular structures must be undertaken by skilled physicians who are aware of all possibilities. I have already discussed blood around the eye. Blood in the eye is called a *hyphema.* It often results from a blunt injury to the eye resulting from such things as a punch, a ball hitting the eye, a seed thrown at the eye, a rubber band snapping into the eye, or a rock thrown at the eye. This is just a sampling of some situations that can occur in life. A young patient of mine while attempting to play the drums too vigorously, poked the drumsticks into his eyes causing a hyphema and a retinal problem.

Since a hyphema can be a common consequence of a contusion injury to the eye, it deserves special mention.

1 – Prognosis for recovery of good visual acuity depends on the extent of the blood level present in the anterior chamber at the time of the examination, and whether the posterior pole or retina has also been affected.

2 – Prognosis is guarded if the blood fills the entire anterior space, a so called *eight ball hemorrhage.*

3 – Blood in a closed space in the front of the eye, can cause pain, and elevate the eye pressure. If this occurs the patient will complain of nausea and even vomit. This condition of pressure elevation is called *secondary glaucoma* and can result from a contusion injury to the eye. Red blood cells act as particulate matter blocking up the drainage system or filter in the eye. If the hemorrhage blocks the pupil making visualization of the posterior part of the eye difficult, ultrasound can be used to rule out a retinal detachment and the possibility of an intraocular foreign body. Hyphemas are designated by how much blood is in the anterior chamber or space. The

level of blood is described in percentages, i.e., ten percent, etc. The doctor records the level in front of the iris in a diagram in the child's chart. As the blood level regresses, changes can be noted in the chart diagram.

Instructions given to patients for follow up care varies with each physician depending on their experience. In my office I preferred to do the following:

1- The child is placed on bed rest with bathroom privileges.

2- There is no patching, since patching often make children more apprehensive. It is important for them to be calm. Sedation is not generally necessary, unless there is a large hyphema and the child is unruly and lacks understanding.

3-During the rest period the eyes should not be used for reading or watching television and subdued lighting is preferred. The aim is to relax the eyes as much as possible since the iris of the eye once traumatized can rebleed between the second and the sixth day following injury.

4 – I also requested that parents keep friends and family out of the child's room to minimize distraction and hyperactivity.

As the blood clears, without a rebleed or pressure in the eye, vision returns to normal. Parents are encouraged to schedule routine follow-ups to check for the possibility of late onset secondary glaucoma years later.

Eye trauma which results in a fracture of the bone around the eye, called the *orbit,* is also not uncommon. In children, orbital fractures may occur from a fall, a baseball thrown from close range hitting the eye, a handle bar injury related to a fall off the bicycle, and less frequently because of seat belts, a car accident.

If the diagnostic scan shows a fracture in the floor of the orbit without facial fractures, the eye plastic physician is called in to correct the problem. If there are associated facial fractures a surgical team is usually required.

Linear fractures that are not initially considered problematic should also be followed for the possibility of a later complaint of double vision and the appearance of limitation of upward gaze. If this occurs it is most likely due to incarceration of orbital tissue in the fracture in the orbital floor. This situation usually warrants surgical intervention. Without these previously mentioned symptoms, orbital floor fractures will heal leaving no permanent sequelae.

CHAPTER XIII

CONGENITAL DISEASES THE ROLE THEY PLAY IN VISION PROBLEMS

Children who have a normal birth history and a normal appearance to their eyes externally, can at times be found to have poor vision. How can this happen? How does the eye physician determine the reason for this unfortunate situation? Many congenital diseases show signs of pathology in the back of the eye or retina, which are not visible to the ordinary observer. Special noninvasive tests can be performed to gauge the health of the retinal cells. One such test is the electroretinogram. This test measures the electric response of the retina to light flashes. If the doctor feels that the retina has unusual deposits or coloration changes in the *macula* or reading center of the eye, a *fluoresein angiogram* can even be performed on a small child. This test is performed with the use of a dye that is injected into a vein in the arm. This vegetable dye travels into the retinal circulation in twelve seconds. Pictures are taken of the back of the eye once the dye perfuses the retina. This test enables the doctor to gain valuable information. If these tests are normal and the so called film in the camera, the retina, is not at fault, a cat scan and mri can be scheduled to rule out pathology in the brain and optic nerves.

A simple test that should always be part of information gathering, along with the electroretinogram is the color vision test. The retinal cells that are responsible for reading vision are called *cone cells*. A congenital disease called cone dysfunction can be detected through information gained by testing for color vision problems. These children have shaky eyes or *nystagmus*, as well as decreased vision. It is important to differentiate this condition from more serious retinal diseases, because cone dysfunction has a better prognosis for vision. Parents can be assured that the nystagmus in this case will lessen with time. The condition does not cause blindness. These children have a normal peripheral field. In addition most of them can function normally in the regular school system.

Albinism or lack of pigment in the iris is another inherited disorder. Unlike the diseases that affect the back of the eye, this condition can present in the front of the eye. Ocular albinism is a sex linked disorder affecting primarily males. The child's mother's eyes should be examined as well. In albinism a flashlight directed toward the normally pigmented iris of the eye shines through easily--it transilluminates. This is because there is insufficient pigment in the iris to prevent the light from entering the eye. In addition, the back of the eye may have decreased pigment, resulting in decreased central vision and abnormal movement of the eyes or nystagmus. Albinism can be divided into three types: complete, incomplete, or partial. Your eye doctor will base her diagnosis on the following information: a careful history and eye examination, the findings on the special test called an electroretinogram, and a color vision test. Complete albinism is also inherited. Consequently, other members of the family need to be examined as well. Patients with complete albinism can present with "shaky eyes" (pendular nystagmus) and poor vision, 20/200 or less. The macula in these patients is weak.

CHAPTER XIV

TESTING FOR POSSIBLE BLINDNESS AT BIRTH

It is difficult to test vision in a newborn. Often unfounded statements that lack true scientific fact are made which cause emotional hardship to parents. Vision is charged with emotion. "Something is wrong." "Does my baby see?" Fortunately, those words are not heard often but when the doctor is confronted with this question she should first establish good communication with the parent, and discuss the baby's eye exam. Basic methods are used in testing visual acuity. Essentially the following steps occur: observation by the examiner, fixation of the infant on an interested object, i.e., a toy, fixation of the infant on a flashlight, and watching if the baby will follow the light. Other techniques can be tried to assess vision depending on the age of the infant. As previously mentioned, a one month old baby is considered a neonate. The doctor can use an optokinetic drum to assess his vision. While the drum is rotated in front of the baby, the doctor observes the eyes for signs of nystagmus or shaky movement. This is a positive sign that the infant has vision. A positive response recorded when the stripes on the drum are made smaller and closer together means that the infant has better visual acuity.

There are subtle signs that a parent should be aware of when the infant is in the crib. Does the newborn notice toys in the crib that are placed in front of him? Does she play with her fingers or toes? Is there an awareness of faces as they crowd over the crib? Part of an eye exam as we have mentioned is getting a good history.

Because visual assessment with the optokinetic drum is not always easy to obtain, further tests are used to provide additional information. A very useful test to determine a positive visual response in this age group is the reaction of the pupil to light directed into the eye. If both pupils constrict equally, this is considered a positive sign for vision. This test shows that the retina, the optic nerve, (or cable to the brain from the eye), and the optic tract (cerebral connections) are functioning on the side that the light is directed. If the pupil does not constrict when light is directed toward the eye, this is considered a negative sign which has poor visual prognosis.

Thus far we have emphasized how important it is for parents to try to assess vision early in the infant's life. Besides the E game, and pictures in a linear presentation there are other tests available that can be tried in older children. Isolated pictures are easier to recognize for preschool children. This test however, does not satisfactorily eliminate a suspicious case of amblyopia Your doctor arrives at this diagnosis after considering all these facts 1- family history, birth history, medical history, growth and development, and finally a thorough ocular examination.

CHAPTER XV

AMBLYOPIA

This subject is a very important one and often misunderstood. The term "lazy eye" often used by individuals stems from the generally held notion that the lack or loss of vision comes from not using one or both eyes. As we have discussed, there are conditions which preclude light from entering the eye. This reduction in light prevents the macula from developing properly. Congenital cataracts, droopy eye lids, eye turns or strabismus, and tumors in or on the eye can all contribute to the loss of sight in the eye afflicted with the condition. Amblyopia most commonly results in cases of misalignment of one or both eyes. The patient sees two objects at the same time, a condition called diplopia or double vision. The brain will shut off or suppress one unclear image in its attempt to see only one object. The stronger eye or dominate eye has a clearer image, whereas the misaligned eye may have intermittent vision or blurred vision and continues to be cerebrally suppressed, resulting in deepening amblyopia.

Amblyopia can also result from a difference in refraction between both eyes. For example, a child can be born with *myopia* or nearsightedness in one eye and *hyperopia* or far sightedness in the other eye. This causes the brain to have two different image sizes. Diplopia can result if there is a greater than 30% disparity between the two images.

A difference in refraction between eyes is very common. Often it goes undiagnosed until the patient develops an eye turn. Lacking sensory stimulation, the weaker visual eye turns in while the dominant stronger eye suppresses the image of the turned in eye. This results in a "lazy eye" or amblyopia. Other visual problems may exist which do not present as an eye turn. These are picked up during preschool testing or in the pediatrician's office. Parents are not always aware of vision problems in their children. A child never complains if she has one good eye. The degree of difference between the refraction of each eye that is necessary to produce a lazy eye depends on the child's specific type of refractive problem.

After reading about amblyopia and how difficult it is to detect and cure it, parents should have gained new resolve not to give up the struggle too soon with the therapy in difficult cases. In reality, loss of an eye can change the direction of a child's life. VISION LOSS CAN BE PREVENTED. Parents should do the following: 1-obtain a good family history; 2-schedule routine eye exams with an ophthalmologist at three, five, seven and nine years of age. These are the formative growth ages for a child's eye; 3-be aware of symptoms such as squinting, head positions that appear unnatural, sitting close to the television, holding books too close, closing or favoring one eye, eyes that are unsteady or move funny, tilting the head back in order for the eyelid to be higher than the pupil; and 4- If eyes do not appear symmetrical in size or shape, it could present a refractive difference which should be checked out.

I have often heard the complaint. "My child can see the blackboard but has trouble seeing notes at the piano". This type of problem can result from having astigmatism. These children have difficulty recognizing if the note is on the line or between the lines.

Finally, if you are told by the pediatrician's office or the school nurse that the vision test showed a difference between the two eyes but together they were 20/20 AND THAT'S OK, DO NOT ACCEPT THIS AS NORMAL. This child should have an eye exam. Eyes, as I have discussed, are usually symmetrical. If they are not, why not? A small difference can mean the existence of amblyopia in one eye due to a small eye turn unappreciated by the parent.

CHAPTER XVI

VISUAL ACUITY – EXPECTATIONS AT A GIVEN AGE

The visual acuity chart is presented as an aid to understanding what your child's level of vision should potentially be at a given age. [4]

LEVEL OF VISUAL ACUITY	METHOD OF TESTING
From birth to approx. 1 mo. Range is 20/50-20/100	Method of testing often objective and with use of rotating drum
From approx. 1 mo. to 1 yr. vision is better than 20/50	Same method of testing as above.
From 1 to 3 yrs. visual acuity is better than 20/50 and can be 20/20	Method of testing, picture cards, E game, find objects

As the child grows and the eye also grows, a difference of only one line between eyes can be very significant. This difference could be a sign of amblyopia in the weaker

[4] Helvaston, Eugene, Ellis, Forest; Pediatric Ophthalmology Practice; Mosby, 1980

eye. An ophthalmologist will rule out the presence or absence of lazy eye. If necessary corrective lenses can reduce the difference in image size and prevent the development of what eye doctors call “anisometropic amblyopia”.

From three years to five years of age or preschool years vision in normal eyes not needing corrective lenses is 20/30 plus. Vision testing becomes easier both for the parent and child. Children of average intelligence can be taught to respond accurately to the E card. Today, most children are taught to know their numbers and letters before they enter kindergarten. They often prefer to be tested with the Snellen chart and not the E cards. Eyes are tested separately with an occluder held over each eye until the child reads the smallest line. Children at this age can also be tested for depth perception with a test called the *Titmus Test*. Polaroid glasses are placed over the child’s eyes. Both eyes are open, not covered during this exam. Normally the patient will notice that some pictures pop out or stand out. Young children are asked to touch the animals that stick out. If they can see nine out of nine stereoscopic pictures, their vision in each eye is usually better than 20/40. This test is a useful guide to parents who ask, “Can my child read with his present vision?” The depth perception test is performed at reading distance and is by its very nature a close up exam. It provides the doctor with useful information regarding reading vision.

In school age children vision is 20 /25 plus in normal eyes that do not need glasses. The Snellen chart is used to test their vision as it is used for adults. If children are referred to an eye doctor because of headaches or difficulty with reading, they will have a dilated exam in order for the eye doctor to get an accurate refraction and examine the retina or back of the eye. The most common age for children to receive their first pair of glasses is around nine years of age.

As previously stated, vision problems are inherited. Therefore, if a parent has worn glasses since childhood it is very likely that her child or one of her children will also wear corrective lenses. Preparing your child for the eventuality allows for greater acceptance. Parents should support the benefits of glasses and not allow their children to make a choice based solely on appearance or peer pressure. When asked, "Should my child wear glasses all the time or part time in school?" the answer depends on the kind of refractive problem the child has. The following is a rough guide:

1- If your child is wearing glasses to correct a lazy eye the glasses are worn all the time. Usually patching of the good or stronger eye is also recommended. Your eye doctor will establish a schedule to be followed depending on the age of your child and the seriousness of the amblyopia.

2 – If your child is wearing glasses for severe or moderate nearsightedness, glasses should be worn throughout the day. Without clear vision your child may not see the approaching individual in the school yard. Clear vision is a form of protection for an innocent child. During my career, I have found that children who are very nearsighted experience sensory deprivation without glasses. They are not tuned into their environment, appear shy and reluctant to engage in activities with other children. As stated, children who have

high myopia should avoid body contact sports such as football where they might incur head trauma.

3 – Normal vision is a term that is used frequently to calm parents' fears that their child is not in danger of a vision problem. At times it is misused. To the eye doctor it simply implies 20/20 uncorrected, good binocularity, and normal color vision. These children can perform all tasks. The term normal vision should not be applied if vision is good in one eye and not the other. As previously mentioned, these patients may have decreased vision in an eye because of an eye turn. These children have no binocularity because they are using only one eye. Despite this handicap, they have little functional impairment. They appear to live normal lives. They use accessory clues to aid them when they are confronted with depth perception situations. For example, a shadow helps them determine how far a chair is from the wall, bigger objects are closer, smaller ones are further away. It is still important for children to understand their visual limitations. They will then select the proper sport to play, thereby reducing their frustrations. They will understand why they can't park their car as well as their friends. The selection of an occupation can also be affected by lacking good stereopsis.

The difficulties with night vision while driving has been an ongoing concern both for parents and teenage patients. A driver's license can be obtained with only 20/60 vision in the best corrected eye. I do not feel that teenagers should drive at night with this type of vision. These patients lack good depth perception even on a clear day. Night driving poses a problem with headlight glare. Glare causes the pupils to constrict and the depth of focus shortens. This is contrary to the normal driver's distant gaze. All of these factors compound the lack of good visual acuity and place the teenager at risk to auto accidents.

OPTOKINETIC DRUM

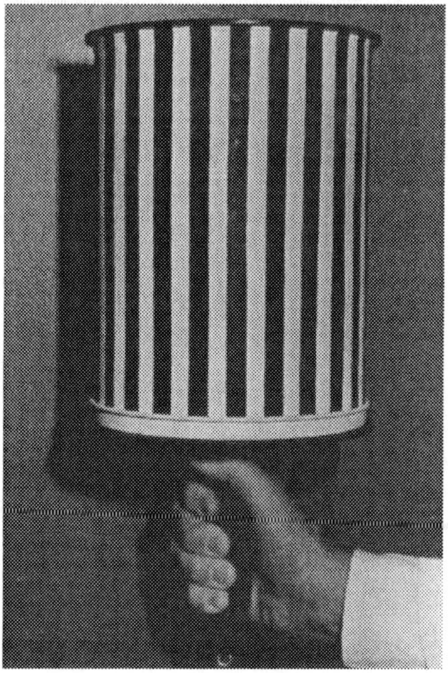

Used to test Infant's Vision

CHAPTER XVII

LEGAL BLINDNESS

This term can be seen on forms to designate a patient's visual acuity level when there is a question of visual handicap or limited vision. It means that a child or individual has a visual acuity of 20/200 or less in the better eye and a limited field of 20 degrees or less in the better eye as determined by a visual field test. This designation is used by agencies to determine eligibility for aid, or school and job placement. It is used to decide whether to give patients special consideration with regard to home assistance, travel arrangements, and even taxes. Legal blindness is not a medical term. It should not provide the patient an opportunity to lack motivation and thereby lose direction in life. It is important to remember that even with limited eyesight the patient can perform normally and have a productive occupation.

I have discussed terms designating types of vision as well as limitation of vision. I have not mentioned the denial of vision or *conversion hysteria*. This is a rare occurrence but can happen even in children. During the eye exam the child refuses to acknowledge recognizing objects or seeing the lines on the eye chart. The eye doctor uses different tests, such as the Titmus test, red-green glasses and visual field test, to determine the truth that the patient is feigning lack of vision. There is frequently a reluctance on the part of the child to see, often based on underlying psychological problems or difficulties at home. My patient was unable to accept or "see" the impending separation of her parents. During the eye exam, I ask parents to leave the room. The titmus fly test is helpful in proving the existence of normal vision. These patients also give inappropriate answers while attempting to see the Snellen Chart. A visual field test should be performed if the patient is old enough. Once the diagnosis is certain the doctor will guide the parents in their attempt through patience and understanding to reveal the underlying emotional issues confronting their child. At times counseling is necessary. Conversion hysteria is self-limiting and will disappear without visual loss once the emotional problem is corrected.

CHAPTER XVIII

PRESCRIPTION GLASSES AND CONTACT LENSES

How does the eye physician determine the proper prescription for children younger than five years of age?

Special testing methods such as a pinhole will quickly tell the physician if visual acuity is correctable with lenses or contacts. Dilating drops are necessary when cooperation is not forthcoming and consistency on the vision test is not accurate. With the use of a streak light from a *retinoscope*, the instrument the doctor holds in her hand, plus loose lenses, she is able to arrive at the proper prescription. At times, in the case of a young patient, two sessions may be necessary. The first exam is designed to "meet and greet" your doctor and become acquainted. Children older than six years of age can be tested with the aid of a *phoropter*, an instrument placed in the front of the patient's face, as they read the eye chart. Dilating drops are usually not necessary for this type of testing.

Putting the patient at ease and making the visit enjoyable is of primary importance. The doctor may elect to use dilating drops that are not harmful. They work quickly to enlarge the pupil in order to provide the viewer with "a good reflex or look in". The affect of the drops is not long lasting, but can cause temporary sensitivity to light. Dark glasses offered to the child after refraction makes him more comfortable for the trip home.

Glasses are usually prescribed in the following cases:

1. Nearsighted patients with a distance vision, without correction, of less than 20/50. Board size print is 20/40. In other words, if the child's vision is weaker than 20/50, glasses are necessary in order that the child be able to see the board from any seat in the room. In addition, children are asked to wear their glasses in school all the time, for reading as well as distance, to ensure continuity of vision from far to near, so that he will not miss anything in the classroom. It is important to note that wearing glasses throughout the day does NOT contribute to weakening of the child's vision or a dependency on his glasses. The only dependency he might find is for clear vision.

2. Very far sighted patients who are not comfortable reading and complain of headaches. In this group, the problem with vision is not easily discovered. They appear to be able to see distance objects comfortably. While driving with their parents, they can read license plates and signs. Yet, in school, they tend to have difficulty staying focused on close activities, such as reading books. To read for a prolonged period of time requires accommodation, focusing at near, which is neces-

sary when one reads. This effort can be tiring for very far sighted children because they have to expend energy when trying to focus on the printed page for any period of time. In addition, these children are easily distracted because they are usually gazing out the window, which is their far point, or comfort point. Teachers tend to describe these children as hyperactive and they are not generally good students. When the doctor gives a prescription to correct this far sightedness, it is advisable that the child wear her glasses throughout the day. In so doing, she becomes a better reader and consequently, a better student. Generally, these children are compliant and happy with their prescription.

If a child is found to be far sighted, but considered by the doctor to be a borderline case for an actual prescription, a schedule for follow-up visits is necessary. Routine visits every six months are scheduled in order to rule out so-called "re fractive esotropia". Parents will recognize this condition as a turning in of one or both eyes, especially when the child reads. Glasses prescribed at this time will usually correct the turn and can prevent amblyopia or "lazy eye".

3. Astigmatism. This is a term used to designate a flattening of the cornea, the shiny part of the eye, or an irregular surface to the eye, which causes a

blurred image and consequently, reduced visual acuity. Many infants are born with astigmatism, which is lessened as the eye matures and may not be present after the age of four. If astigmatism is present in one eye and that eye has a significant blurred image, the brain will select the clear image, thus suppressing or "shutting off" the weaker eye. This visual weakness can induce a condition called refractive amblyopia in a young child. This type of amblyopia is caused by a significant astigmatism in the visually weaker eye. If discovered early, amblyopia can be prevented with glasses. Patching may also be necessary to break up the dominance (if longstanding) of the stronger eye. All these situations are carefully assessed on an individual basis. The goal is always to obtain the best possible vision for the patient. If vision is slowly declining, amblyopia should be suspected.

4. Are bifocal glasses indicated? They are generally prescribed to reduce the deviation in an eye that is turning in when the patient is reading. This condition is called "accommodative esotropia". After retinoscopy, and a dilated refraction, the eye physician determines that the addition of plus lenses or so-called "adds," as in a bifocal, appears to reduce the eye turn significantly at near, she will then prescribe a bifocal. This bifocal should be of such height in the corrective lenses that it bisects the pupil. Since these glasses are worn throughout

the day, the bifocal could present problems with walking downstairs, or blurring distance if the glasses are not fitted properly. If the glasses pose a problem to the child, the bifocal segment can be lowered to the edge of the pupil. The prescription originally provided will change as the child grows. Consequently, there is a need for routine follow-ups with your doctor. When the child's refractive power decreases as he matures, the bifocal might be eliminated. Bifocals should never be prescribed to help children read in order to just reduce eye strain. A nearsighted child, or myope, should NEVER be given a bifocal. Children who are myopic have normal magnification at near. Near vision is clear to them at all times. It is their natural strength. If you give children visual support unnecessarily, it weakens their normal focusing power, which we call accommodation. As we age, the power to accommodate naturally weakens. That is why people need reading glasses after a certain age, usually in their forties. In order not to promote changes in their normal accommodation prematurely, children should never be given a crutch for reading. Only in special situations where children have severe visual handicaps, are strong or so-called plus bifocals prescribed. These children, who may also have multiple handicaps, do function better at near with the aid of high magnification. Finally, as I have also seen, a bifocal should never be situated at the top of the lens.

5. *Contact Lenses.* When should they be prescribed? Who should wear them? Are they safe? Children who are nearsighted and prefer contacts over glasses, are good candidates if they are old enough to understand how to care for them and maintain good hygiene. The age at which they receive contact lenses will depend on their own maturity and the parents' willingness to arrange for regular vision check ups. The average age in my office was twelve years. Some parents, who are unhappy with spectacles, try to convince the doctor to allow the child to wear contact lenses as soon as the patient receives her first prescription. The child is usually nine years of age at the time of her first prescription. A young child loses motivation early and therefore tends to revert back to glasses when she would most benefit from the use of contact lenses, i.e., as an adolescent.

Patients should be allowed to wear contact lenses in sports, such as basketball and tennis. Contact lenses worn on the field, such as in baseball, football and soccer, are controversial. Patients complain of dust getting under their lenses or losing them altogether. Safety glasses in these cases are a better choice. Contact lenses are especially helpful for therapeutic reasons, namely to build vision in patients who need a correction for high myopia in one eye. A contact lens over the weaker eye will allow the image size to be more like the stronger eye. As mentioned if there is greater than thirty percent disparity between both eyes, the brain cannot fuse the image or put the two pictures together and blend them into one. Parents are taught how to place the contact lens on a baby's cornea and instructed how to take out the contact lens. Their cooperation enables their child to have a stronger visual outcome and lessens the chance of the weaker eye becoming severely amblyopic.

Contact lenses are also especially useful in patients with an irregular cornea or astigmatism. The specially fitted lens acts to smooth out the uneven cornea, sits in place, and thereby creates a clearer image. Glasses in these patients may never sit properly, thereby losing their effectiveness.

Aphakia is a special condition, which when it exists, necessitates corrective lenses or contact lenses in order for the patient to see. The term is derived from the Greeks, meaning: a-without; phakos-lens, in other words, without your own natural lens that you had in your eye at birth. Aphakia occurs in children who develop cataracts, either congenitally or from trauma, and need cataract surgery. In adults, cataract surgery is performed with intraocular implants, which are placed in the eye at the time of the surgery. These implants take the place of their own natural lens, thus allowing these patients to see well following surgery. In children, depending on the age of the child and condition of the eye, cataracts are removed and implantation of lenses may be delayed for a future operation or in some cases not possible. These patients receive glasses or contact lenses to restore their vision.

At this point, it is relevant to discuss some general facts concerning cataracts in children. Congenital cataracts cause visual deprivation since they block light from entering the eye and thereby reduce stimulation to the foveal cells which are located in the retina, the film in the so-called camera of the eye. In this case, the retina is not able to develop normally and consequently visual acuity is compromised. Congenital cataracts may account for as much as twenty-three percent of all childhood cataracts. [5] These cataracts are also considered a dominant trait in the genetic makeup of a child.

I have mentioned how important family history becomes when an eye problem is evaluated. This is one such example. Cataracts in children are often associated with other systemic, or body involvement diseases. The pediatrician will be consulted in connection with a finding of congenital cataract(s). Blood tests for glucose, serum calcium and phosphorus, plus a urine analysis are required. In addition, a genetic urine screen, used to rule out metabolic diseases is necessary.

---

[5] Helveston, Eugene, Ellis, Forrest; Pediatric Ophthalmology Practice; Mosby, 1980

CHAPTER XIX

FREQUENTLY ASKED QUESTIONS

1. What is Keratoconus? The cornea has a cone like shape, hence the term. This increased curvature causes a central corneal thinning. At times, the condition progresses, causing scars to form in the center of the cornea. Vision is reduced secondary to clouding of the cornea and astigmatism. Special contact lenses, which are semi soft or hard, can improve vision. If the condition deteriorates, the cornea may perforate. Corneal transplant surgery has been successful in correcting this serious problem. This condition requires an evaluation by a specially trained eye physician, fellowship trained in corneal diseases and surgery.

2. What does it mean when my baby appears to have a fully dilated pupil in one eye, or an absence of the colored part of the eye, the *iris*?

   This is called *aniridia*, lacking an iris. These babies may also have a shaky eye or nystagmus, and appear light sensitive. When examined, they have poor vision, 20/200 in the affected eye. They may also have cataracts and immature development of the fovea in the back of the eye. Patients with these findings need to be followed for glaucoma in later life. Fortunately, many cases of aniridia are not as visually incapacitating. They are however, familial and autosomal dominant. This means that families pass this trait on to their offspring. Thankfully, many do have good vision.

3. What does it mean when my baby has different colored irises? The iris is lighter on one eye than the other. The pigmented iris is the normal eye, blue being the absence of pigment. This condition can be inherited. It is not associated with poor vision and is cosmetic in nature. If however, there are missing areas of pigment on one eye, or sectors missing as compared with the other eye, these patients should be followed for changes in eye pressure and possible glaucoma in later life.

4. What is albinism and how does it affect the eye? Albinism is a congenital disease. Patients lack pigment in the iris of their eyes. Some forms of albinism also show signs of loss of pigment in the skin and hair as well. In children who manifest ocular albinism, nystagmus or shaky movement of the eye, may also be present. In these instances, poor vision and photophobia, or light sensitivity, may also result. The degree of visual loss parallels the lack of pigment in the back of the eye, the foveal area. Ocular albinism is sex

linked and occurs primarily as mentioned in males. [6] I have stated that the fovea is the important part of the retina responsible for good central vision. Lacking pigment in the macula or fovea, the retinal cells do not mature properly and this results in loss of visual discrimination. The ophthalmologist determines the presence of ocular albinism in patients who have suggestive signs with the aid of a light beam from the slit lamp, shining into the white of the eye and the iris. The white area is called the sclera. In cases of ocular albinism, the light appears to shine straight through the eye or transilluminates as mentioned previously.

5. What is color blindness? Does a failure on the office color test mean color blindness? The answer is no. The test used to determine color blindness or deficiency is called an Ishihara Test. The patient is asked to identify objects or patterns. In very small children who may not recognize the shape or object, I ask them to trace the pattern that they see with a finger. The booklet is held close, which of course necessitates the presence of normal vision for near. In older children, the Farnsworth Test can be used. Many patients have told me that color vision was not always tested in a previous eye exam. This is because color defi-

---

[6] Helveston, Eugene, Ellis, Forrest, Pediatric Ophthalmology Practice; Mosby, 1980

ciencies, or defects, are very rare. In patients who have positive findings, such as nystagmus, iris hypopigmentation, or decreased pigmentation, poor vision, and a family history of color vision problems, it becomes essential to conduct a careful color vision exam. Parents can request a color vision test, if their small child has been unable to recognize his colors. Approximately eight percent of white males have a red/green color deficiency. [7] Both colors present with a different hue or saturation to the observer. They then equate the different color as the red or green that the normal person perceives. Women are less affected with loss of color discrimination. Only one percent may be color deficient. Too much emphasis is placed on color deficiency. Parents often redirect their children toward future job opportunities wrongly, based upon this imperfection of nature. Blue/yellow color deficiency is even more rare than red/green.

Complete color blindness is extremely rare. It is inherited and may be present in the first year of an infant's life, unfortunately also associated with nystagmus, light sensitivity and poor vision.

6. Why does my child need muscle exercises or convergence exercises? Do they improve read-

---

[7] Helveston, Eugene, Ellis, Forrest, Pediatric Ophthalmology Practice; Mosby, 1980

ing? If after a thorough eye examination your physician determines that there is a latent turning of the eyes when fatigued, glasses or convergence exercises might be indicated. Exercises in the case of out turning to build so called convergence tonus increases the power of the eye to maintain focus on a near object for a normal period of time. These are called convergence exercises. The child is instructed to focus on a near finger with fixed finger positioned behind it. The near finger is brought closer and closer to the nose. With these repeated exercises the ability to fuse at near will strengthen, which lessens fatigue at near. Parents maintain that their children become better readers. They stay at the task longer. The need for convergence exercises, as stated, depends on the existence of an underlying muscle problem. If it does not exist, these exercises are fruitless. I have found that most of these children who received so-called exercises, from ancillary centers, did not show improvement in their reading skills, nor did they have a muscle problem, therefore not needing the exercises in the first place. Fusional ability, or the coming together of images into one, will lessen fatigue while reading, but truly does not improve the child's reading ability or comprehension. In certain refractive problems, glasses plus exercises will help. Your eye physician will guide you.

7. Should my child wear reading glasses to become a better reader? Most children have good focusing power at the reading distance of 14-16 inches and would not benefit from receiving a reading prescription. Myops, or nearsighted children, see best at near without glasses. For them, there is no effort expended at near. Young hyperops also can easily focus up close. Their need for correction can exist if they demonstrate above average far sightedness. In these cases, correction can be helpful to reduce fatigue far and near.

There are moments when, as physicians, we are not purists about the need for reading glasses. This is true if a parent relates a story of a child unable to keep up with the class. In these cases, I have found that a prescription with a light magnification is useful while he is reading, especially in an early young reader who needs to gain confidence as he matures. There are times when reading glasses can be harmful if the prescription is too strong. This is because the prescription eliminates the need for the eye to accommodate or focus, thereby weakening normal accommodation, which is controlled by involuntary smooth muscles activated cerebrally and not controlled by the reader. After the use of strong unnecessary lenses, the child is unable to see anything at near once he removes his glasses. This is due to relaxation of the smooth muscles involved with focusing through a prescription that is too strong.

Young readers who stop and go and lose their place on the page can be helped with a ruler or bookmark under the sentence they are reading to encourage them to stay on the line and not read down the page. All other gimmicks are just that – gimmicks.

8. Should children wear sunglasses? At what age should they start wearing them?

We live in a world of increasing concern about the environment. The days of sun worship are over. Dermatologists advise us to use sunscreen in order to prevent the harmful rays of the sun from damaging our children's skin. Less publicity and concern has been given to preventing the sun from its toxic effect on children's eyes.

Children have larger pupils than adults. This anatomical situation allows more natural light to enter their eyes. They often appear light sensitive. Children who are blonder or have red hair are most vulnerable to the penetrating affect of the rays that enter their eyes. The iris color is also important. Blue, greenish brown or light hazel eyes have less pigment in their iris. Consequently, the iris in these eyes does not contract as well as in brown eyes. Blue eyes in toddlers and young children always appear dilated to a causal observer. The cumulative effects of sunlight on susceptible eyes may play a part in the increasing number of patients that we now see with the diagnosis of macular degeneration.

I have emphasized "prevention" throughout this book as a key word. I have always believed that all children, starting with toddlers, should be protected from the sun's harmful rays with the aid of proper sunglasses. These should fit well, be made with polycarbonate safety lenses, and tinted green or brown, not black. A black tint can reduce a child's threshold for normal luminosity, thereby making the child light sensitive to ordinary light when the glasses are removed. Children's sunglasses should have a label attached, stating that the lenses include U. V. protection.

CHAPTER XX

READING PROBLEMS OR DYSLEXIA

Dyslexia is a Greek word which means difficulty (dys) with words (lexia). We hear this term used frequently by the public who label children as dyslexic. Children with this condition have difficulty with processing their visual stimuli. The eye transmits nerve impulses to the brain. The brain must then process these impulses. Because clues in word recognition are transmitted through the eyes to the brain, the eyes have been targeted as the offending agent. In fact, studies have shown that eye defects do not cause reversals of letters, words or numbers. Most ophthalmologists feel that patients who present with the possible diagnosis of dyslexia should be evaluated by a team consisting of pediatricians, ear, nose and throat doctors, audiologists, neurologists and psychiatrists. Those who wish to treat patients by means of visual training, such as muscle exercises, ocular pursuit and glasses, or so-called neurological organizational training, balance board or perceptual training, cause economic hardship for parents and may delay the truly necessary care needed for these children. Many dyslexics have successful lives, their only weakness being poor spelling and slow reading.

The role of the ophthalmologist in problems related to reading difficulties has been reviewed. Essentially, it is to provide a thorough, comprehensive evaluation of the child's eye. If there is a refractive problem, provide proper corrective glasses. Eye exams should begin at age three, unless there is prematurity, in which case eye exams should start at three months of age and follow up with a retina specialist. If there is a muscle imbalance correct it with glasses if necessary, prisms or surgery when indicated. The ophthalmologist must inform parents of the results of the examination. With proper education, a parent can then guard against those practioners who wish to exploit the eyes because of lack of knowledge or for profit.

FINAL REMARKS

This book was inspired by my patients' need for information regarding their children's eye problems. I have attempted to discuss common topics in a straightforward manner. I have not included a thorough review of all eye problems since this is not a textbook. I hope that my readers will use this information to reduce apprehension and anxiety with regard to their children's eye care. Perhaps the most important message to be gained from this book is that the eye is a very complicated and delicate organ

Knowledge of potential problems with your child's eyes is the key to early detection. Through good, professional care, vision can be restored and maintained. Value your eyes. Protect them. Care for them. And, above all, do not be casual or dismissive when it comes to vision. Vision, unfortunately, can easily slip away. Do not let it happen to you or your loved ones.

GLOSSARY

Accommodation – is a neurologic process, not voluntary, which causes the power of the lens to increase and thicken in order to focus at near.

Amblyopia – reduced vision or poor vision in an eye most often due to deviation or misalignment of any, as in strabismus. It can result from other causes, such as a cataract.

Anisometropia – the refractive states of the two eyes are different, i.e., one is near sighted, the other far sighted.

Astigmatism – is an optical condition commonly described as a "lack of smoothness to the cornea", thereby causing a blurred image.

Cataract – opacity in the lens of the eye.

Chalazion – bump on eyelid from an infection in the glands of the eyelids.

Convergence Insufficiency – condition in which the eyes fail to fuse the image at a near point.

Diplopia – double vision.

Epicanthus – the skin fold on either side of the nose.

Esotropia – eye turns in as patient looks straight ahead.

Exotropia – eye turns out as patient looks straight ahead.

Glaucoma – abnormal elevation of pressure in the eye causing damage to the optic nerve in the back of the eye.

Nystagmus – an involuntary back and forth or jerky movement of the eye (there are many kinds).

Orbit – bony socket which holds the eye.

Pseudostrabismus (false strabismus) – is a condition in which the eyes appear crossed but are perfectly aligned.

Ptosis – droopy eyelid.

Stereopsis – depth perception.

Strabismus – a condition in which the eyes are not directed together, thereby not focusing the object of regard into one picture.

Suppression – the condition in which an image of one eye is essentially blocked and not perceived as the child looks at an object. This condition leads to amblyopia and loss of depth perception.